YOUR KNOWLEDGE HAS VALUE

- We will publish your bachelor's and master's thesis, essays and papers

- Your own eBook and book - sold worldwide in all relevant shops

- Earn money with each sale

Upload your text at www.GRIN.com and publish for free

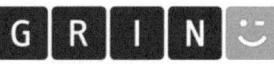

Bibliographic information published by the German National Library:

The German National Library lists this publication in the National Bibliography; detailed bibliographic data are available on the Internet at http://dnb.dnb.de .

This book is copyright material and must not be copied, reproduced, transferred, distributed, leased, licensed or publicly performed or used in any way except as specifically permitted in writing by the publishers, as allowed under the terms and conditions under which it was purchased or as strictly permitted by applicable copyright law. Any unauthorized distribution or use of this text may be a direct infringement of the author s and publisher s rights and those responsible may be liable in law accordingly.

Imprint:

Copyright © 2018 GRIN Verlag
Print and binding: Books on Demand GmbH, Norderstedt Germany
ISBN: 9783668637733

This book at GRIN:

https://www.grin.com/document/412263

Patrick Kimuyu

Aspects of Normal Ageing and Their Relationship with the Development of Disability, Iatrogenic Illness and Geriatric Syndromes

GRIN Verlag

GRIN - Your knowledge has value

Since its foundation in 1998, GRIN has specialized in publishing academic texts by students, college teachers and other academics as e-book and printed book. The website www.grin.com is an ideal platform for presenting term papers, final papers, scientific essays, dissertations and specialist books.

Visit us on the internet:

http://www.grin.com/

http://www.facebook.com/grincom

http://www.twitter.com/grin_com

Aspects of Normal Ageing and Their Relationship with the Development of Disability, Iatrogenic Illness and Geriatric Syndromes

Patrick Kimuyu

Introduction

Over the past decades, scientific inquiry into the phenomenon of aging has produced extensive literature. Of great fascination is the mechanism that underlies aging process. From a biological perspective, aging takes a life course when an individual grows to maturity. During this phase in life, aging is not felt as a remarkable biological course due to the excitement that occurs during young age. However, the ageing coincides with explicit biological changes, especially the aspect of physical decline. It is this phase of ageing that has attracted the interests of both scientists and gerontologists. Scientists are focused on understanding the biology of aging. Biological studies indicate that ageing involves biological pathways such as the regulation of genes, metabolism and cellular signaling (López-Otín et al., 2013; Newgard & Pessin, 2014). These pathways play integral roles in controlling how the human body works including response to infection, stress, as well as recovery from injuries. On the other hand, gerontologists are concerned with the aspects of aging, in order to distinguish normal aging from disease. The task here involves establishing a clear boundary between normal aging and age-related health problems which have, for long, been considered as part of aging. For instance, the association of change in personality, especially during old age has been found to be an independent construct that does not have a significant relationship with normal ageing (National Institute of Health, 2015). In this respect, this paper provides a critical discussion on aspects of normal ageing, when combined with a chronic disease, may contribute to the development of disability, iatrogenic illness and geriatric syndromes, as well as elucidating the nurse's role in limiting this risk. This topic has immense implications to clinical practice. Foremost, ageing is associated with chronic illnesses. Additionally, some aspects of ageing exhibit interplay with chronic illnesses to cause devastating health consequences such as disability, iatrogenic illness and geriatric syndromes. Therefore, nursing care should focus on addressing chronic illnesses, as well as preventing the development of disability, iatrogenic illness and geriatric syndromes. As such, this essay discusses how the combination of normal ageing aspects with chronic illnesses may lead to these adverse health conditions using the case of diabetes.

Impact of Diabetes on Aged Adults

In definition, diabetes is a chronic metabolic disorder that is associated with hyperglycemia (Chentli, Azzoug & Mahgoun, 2015). It is reported to have the highest prevalence and mortality among older adults. As such, Kirkman et al. (2012) cites ageing of the global population as a significant risk factor of diabetes epidemic. Consequently, the combination of ageing with diabetes increases the risk of disability, geriatric syndromes and iatrogenic disease. Evidence indicates that diabetes in old adults leads to geriatric syndromes such as cognitive dysfunction (Punthakee et al., 2012). On the other hand, diabetes in older adults has been found to cause disability due to falls, fractures and visual impairment (Kirkman et al., 2012). Similarly, normal ageing and diabetes increase the risk of iatrogenic disease due to polypharmacy. In most cases, polypharmacy causes drug-disease or drug-drug interactions which result into adverse health outcomes (Onder et al., 2013; Huang et al., 2010).

Ageing and Body Changes

Overall, the mechanisms of ageing are associated to the novel changes that occur in the body, both at cellular and molecular levels. These cause changes in the way tissues, organs and organ systems carry out their biological functions. Therefore, it is possible to elucidate an array of aspects of normal ageing, in order to define their relationship with age-related health problems. In retrospect, there are several aspects of normal ageing, when combined with diabetes, may contribute to the development of disability, iatrogenic illness and geriatric syndromes. Some of these aspects of normal ageing include tissue changes, physical decline, cognitive decline, decreased skeletal strength, visual impairment, and reproductive health decline.

Tissue Changes

Tissue change during ageing is the most explicit aspect of normal ageing that has significant health implications. From a biological perspective, mammalian cells undergo several biological mechanisms that ensure that all tissues have functional cells to carry out their biological functions. Therefore, tissues are rejuvenated with new cells through a constant replacement of the old tissue cells. At the cellular level, several mechanisms underlie the process of cell ageing. This process occurs at different rates depending with the nature and function of the cells involved. As such, cell ageing occurs differently from the ordinary molecular ageing. Ideally, molecular ageing involves a significant decline in cellular activity, as well as structural changes, rather than the replacement of old cells with new ones.

In this context, it is worth elucidating significant tissue changes that are associated with normal ageing. Ordinarily, ageing is known to affect the function of organs, a phenomenon that may increase the risk of chronic illnesses. This explains why chronic illnesses are highly prevalent among the elderly population compared to the other age groups. In most cases, elderly people experience more than one chronic illness. These illnesses are related to other age-related health conditions such as geriatric syndromes and iatrogenic illness.

Hardening of the Blood Vessels

One of the tissue changes with devastating health consequences during the process of ageing is the hardening of the blood vessels. Anatomical studies indicate that ageing is accompanied by changes in the blood vessels. For instance, blood vessels in the heart have been found to lose their elasticity as one grows old. Additionally, fatty deposits accumulate on the coronary blood vessels. This tissue change is of great concern because it increases the risk of heart disease. From a biological perspective, build up of fatty deposits in the blood vessels leads to the formation of plaques, a phenomenon referred to as atherosclerosis. This is the hardening of the arteries which interferes with the laminar flow of blood, especially in the coronary arteries. In adult diabetic patients, the development of atherosclerosis increases the risk of hypertension and other cardiovascular diseases. Evidence from biomedical studies indicates that atherosclerosis serves as the main cause of hypertension, coronary heart disease, heart attack, as well as other cardiovascular conditions. In the elderly, blood vessel tissue changes increases the risk of suffering from cardiovascular diseases. On the other hand, atherosclerosis or rather hypertension is associated with stroke. This explains why most old people are suffering from stroke compared to other populations. Therefore, the combination of this phenomenon with diabetes leads to the development of disability. It is apparent that stroke accounts for a high percentage of disability among the elderly. Global epidemiological data show that stroke is among the chronic conditions that are causing disability (Chappell & Cooke, 2010).

Renal Function Decline

Ageing is also known to influence renal function. Ordinarily, renal function declines with age due to changes in the renal tissue. In most cases, this characteristic decline in renal function raises health concerns, especially in patients with diabetes. Renal failure is one of the complications of diabetes. It has emerged as one of the most challenging health issues among the old diabetic people. Therefore, the combination of renal function decline with diabetes raises concerns among gerontologists. Foremost, renal failure in diabetic patients increases the risk of drug-induced iatrogenic disease. In turn, renal failure increases the incidence of drug-disease, or drug-drug interactions leading to the development of iatrogenic disease. Second, renal failure in diabetic cases leads to catheterization, which in turn increases chances of infection. As a result, treatment for such infections increases the risk of drug-induced iatrogenic disease.

Decreased Elasticity of the Gut Muscles

Finally, changes in the gut tissues during ageing affect the health of old people. Ageing is known to be accompanied by decreased elasticity of the gut muscles. It is also accompanied by a gradual decline in the production of digestive enzymes, as well as gastric secretions that enhance food digestion. These normal changes affect the integrity of the gut, including decrease in food absorption, gastric emptying time and intestinal microbial balance. This is why most old people develop an array of digestive disorders. In the event these normal ageing changes combine with diabetes, the affected people experience an increased risk of iatrogenic disease. Diabetes is associated with metabolic problems including digestion and absorption of food nutrients from the gut. Therefore, the decline in gut function in old people is associated with digestive problems which increase the use of drugs. In turn, drugs used to treat digestive disorders may cause drug-induced iatrogenic disease. In one prospective study, the use of laxatives was found to be associated with falls (Bloch et al., 2010).

Physical Decline

Physical decline is also a significant aspect of normal ageing. Biologically, physical decline is characterized by a gradual decrease in mobility or physical activity. Ageing is usually accompanied by a gradual decrease of muscle activity. As a result, decreased muscle activity, especially skeletal muscles which are involved in movement leads to a slowdown in old age. This aspect of normal ageing demonstrates why people in old age are not as active as they were during their adolescent and early adulthood. In the athletic career, ageing is known to slowdown runners. This is why age is considered as one the main determinants of success in sports competitions. Therefore, physical decline is a key aspect of normal ageing. Unfortunately, occurrences of chronic illnesses during ageing, especially those which affect skeletal muscles' activity have devastating health consequences to the elderly. For instance, the combination of physical decline with diabetes creates a physical challenge to the elderly.

In most cases, diabetes causes physical mobility difficult resulting to disability. Similarly, diabetes related complications such as diabetic foot and neuropathy increase the risk of disability in old people due to the effects of physical decline. Biologically, the rate of bone formation decreases with age. This is why osteoporosis is quite prevalent among people aged over 50 years. Therefore, the combination of physical decline with diabetes may lead to the development of disability among the elderly. In practice, the occurrence of multiple chronic diseases serves as one the key risk factors for iatrogenic disease. Therefore, the treatment of diabetes in old people has been found to exacerbate the development of other chronic conditions. According to Permpongkosol (2011), the use of non-steroidal anti-inflammatory drugs in the treatment of inflammation as it is the case in diabetes and arthritis may precipitate chronic gastric irritation as it is the case with ibuprofen. As a result, the treatment and management of these chronic conditions may lead to the development of iatrogenic disease.

Cognitive Decline

Cognitive decline is another aspect of normal ageing which, when combined with some chronic illnesses may lead to the development of disability. Initially, it was perceived that the occurrence of sudden personality changes such as becoming withdrawn, depressed, or cranky was an aspect of normal ageing. However, extensive studies on this aspect by scientists are revealing the biochemical basis of personality changes in old people (National Institute of Health, 2015). Surprisingly, evidence indicates that personality changes during ageing are attributable to pathological consequences. Based on the results of the Baltimore Longitudinal Study of Aging (BLSA), ageing is accompanied by gradual cognitive changes which are attributable to the loss of brain volume. Therefore, scientists in this study conclude that sudden personality changes during ageing reveals the onset of a mental health disorder. Therefore, gerontologists are concerned with the relationship between cognitive decline during ageing and mental health illnesses. For instance, it is likely that the combination of cognitive decline with diabetes related neuropathy may lead to the development of disability. According to epidemiological evidence, dementia accounts for a significant portion of disability cases during ageing. As reported by Chappell and Cooke (2010), mental impairment serves as one of the leading causes of disability among the elderly.

Visual Impairment

Biologically, ageing is accompanied by a gradual visual decline. As an individual grows old, visual ability decreases, even when there are no other environmental factors. Therefore, visual decline is one of the main aspects of normal ageing. However, this phenomenon may lead to the development of disability when combined with some chronic illnesses. For instance, diabetes has been known to be one of the chronic illnesses whose complications lead to visual impairment or blindness. Over the years, investigations into the biochemical mechanism that underlie the development of retinopathy among diabetic patients have generated significant evidence how this condition develops. In the elderly, who already experience visual decline as a normal process of ageing, the development of diabetes exacerbates visual impairment. In turn, visual impairment is considered as a significant risk factor for disability among the elderly (Chappell & Cooke, 2010).

Sexual Tissue Changes

Ageing is also accompanied by changes of sexual tissues which compromise reproductive health during old age. Biologically, vaginal fluid production decreases with age in women, especially after reproductive age. On the other hand, most men experience sexual tissue atrophy. All these changes in both women and men occur as normal processes during ageing. However, the combination of sexual tissue changes with some chronic illnesses may lead to the development of geriatric syndromes. For instance, some chronic conditions such as diabetes have been found to be associated with urinary incontinence (Chiu, Huang, Wang & Kuo, 2012).

Physiologic Reserve and Function Decline

Physiologic reserve and function decline is a significant aspects of normal ageing (Barzilai, Huffman, Muzumdar & Bartke, 2012). In most cases, geriatric syndromes develop as a result of ageing. One of the most common age related geriatric syndromes is frailty. According to Chen, Mao and Leng (2014), frailty syndrome is common among people aged above 50 years. In other words, frailty emerges as an age related syndrome with its highest incidence among the elderly. Additionally, it is reported that the development of frailty during ageing is attributable to chronic inflammation which occur due to environmental stressors, chronic diseases, metabolic factors, or genetic factors. In retrospect, an array of biomedical studies has explained the relationship between frailty syndrome and normal ageing in old adults. Overall, the pathogenesis of frailty syndrome is associated with chronic inflammation (Collerton et al., 2012; Leng et al., 2011; Ramarathan et al., 2013). Another significant condition that underlies the development of frailty in old people is sarcopenia, a characteristic skeletal mass loss that occur during ageing (Liu et al., 2013).

Impacts of Disability, Geriatric Syndromes and Iatrogenic Illness on Practice

Overall, disability, geriatric syndromes and iatrogenic illness, especially among old adults have significant implications to nursing practice and clinical practice, in general. These conditions are associated with morbidity and mortality. In most cases, physicians and nurses focus on providing treatment and management interventions for chronic illnesses and fail to consider the benefits of addressing some of these age related health outcomes. In the Australian context, nurses have several roles in limiting the risk of co-occurrence of chronic illnesses with iatrogenic disease and geriatric syndromes in old people. First, nurses can prevent the development of geriatric syndromes, disability and iatrogenic disease through ensuring that old people get proper nutrition. In practice, nutrition plays significant roles in preventing chronic illnesses, as well as promoting healthy ageing. Nutrient starvation has adverse health outcomes (Shang et al., 2011). For instance, metabolic changes in diabetic patients, especially the elderly causes impairment of glucose metabolism. Skeletal muscles are not able to utilize glucose for respiration purposes due to insulin resistance which prevent glucose from entering into the cells for the generation of ATP energy. As a result, glucose accumulates in the plasma causing hyperglycemic conditions. Instead, the body oxidizes fatty acids for energy generation. Therefore, nutrition therapy in old people, especially those suffering from diabetes plays a critical role in reducing diabetes complications. According to Kim (2014), nutrition therapy focuses on addressing the nutrition needs of diabetic patients. Among the elderly, nutrition therapy is of paramount importance, especially in promoting healthy living and prevention of diabetes, as well as other chronic metabolic disorders which may increase the risk of geriatric syndromes or disability. Evidence indicates that nutrition therapy has substantial benefits including altering lipid profile and enhancing glycemic control (Andrews et al., 2011). Second, nurses can reduce the adverse health outcomes among the elderly through identifying and addressing iatrogenic disease and geriatric syndromes (Blinderman, 2010). For instance, controlling the use of laxatives in treating digestive disorders in old people can reduce recurring falls (Permpongkosol, 2011). Finally, nurses can prevent the risk of disability, geriatric syndromes and iatrogenic disease through preventing socioeconomic, environmental and biological stressors among old people. This can be achieved through the development of evidence-based nursing interventions, especially those which help to prevent the development of chronic illnesses. It is worth noting that most chronic illnesses such as diabetes, hypertension, heart disease and some cancers can be prevented through lifestyle modification. They are caused by modifiable risk factors. For instance, obesity, which is a risk factor for diabetes, atherosclerosis and cardiovascular diseases, can be controlled through physical activity and prudent dietary regime. Overall, obesity is to blame for most co-morbidities among old people. Therefore, patient education on healthy lifestyle modifications in nursing homes can go a long way in reducing the risk of disability, iatrogenic and geriatric syndromes.

Conclusion

Conclusively, ageing is significant biological process. Biologically, normal ageing is associated to a decline in physiologic reserve, skeletal muscle strength, visual, cognitive, and physical decline. Other tissue changes include deposition of fat in heart vessels, loss of lung tissue elasticity and sexual tissue changes. In some cases, a combination of these aspects of normal ageing lead to the development of disability, geriatric syndromes and iatrogenic disease.

Therefore, this paper offers some recommendations for nurses to enhance health outcomes in old people. First, nurses should ensure that geriatric syndromes are identified and treated as they manage chronic illnesses. Second, they should monitor the nutrition of old people and create awareness to enhance proper nutrition for old adults. Finally, nurses should address socioeconomic, biological and environmental stressors that affect normal ageing.

References

Andrews, R., Cooper, A., Montgomery, A., Norcross, A., Peters, T., Sharp, D.,...Coulman, K. (2011). Diet or diet plus physical activity versus usual care in patients with newly diagnosed type 2 diabetes: the Early ACTID randomised controlled trial. *Lancet, 378,* 129–139.

Barzilai, N., Huffman, D., Muzumdar, R., & Bartke, A. (2012). The critical role of metabolic pathways in aging. *Diabetes, 61,* 1315–1322.

Blinderman, C. D. (2010). Opioids, iatrogenic harm and disclosure of medical error. *J Pain Symptom Manage, 39*(2), 309–313.

Bloch, F., Thibaud, M., Dugue, B., Breque, C., Rigaud, A., & Kemoun, G. (2010). Laxatives as a risk factor for iatrogenic falls in elderly subjects: Myth or reality? *Drugs Aging, 27*(11), 895–901.

Chappell, N., & Cooke, H. (2010). *Age related disabilities - aging and quality of life.* Retrieved from http://cirrie.buffalo.edu/encyclopedia/en/article/189/

Chen, X., Mao, G., & Leng, S. X. (2014). Frailty syndrome: an overview. *Clin Interv Aging, 9,* 433–441. doi: 10.2147/CIA.S45300

Chentli, F., Azzoug, S., & Mahgoun, S. (2015). Diabetes mellitus in elderly. *Indian J Endocrinol Metab., 19*(6), 744–752.

Chiu, A., Huang, M., Wang, C., & Kuo, H. (2012). Prevalence and factors associated with overactive bladder and urinary incontinence in community-dwelling Taiwanese. *TZU chi Medical Journal, 24*(2), 56-60. doi: http://dx.doi.org/10.1016/j.tcmj.2012.03.002

Collerton, J., Martin-Ruiz, C., Davies, K., Hilkens, C., Isaacs, J., Kolenda, C.,...Kirkwood, T. (2012). Frailty and the role of inflammation, immunosenescence and cellular ageing in the very old: cross-sectional findings from the Newcastle 85+ Study. *Mech Ageing Dev., 133,* 456–466.

Huang, E., Karter, A., Danielson, K., Warton, E., & Ahmed, A. (2010). The association between the number of prescription medications and incident falls in a multi-ethnic population of adult type-2 diabetes patients: the Diabetes and Aging Study. *J Gen Intern Med., 25,* 141–146.

Kim, H. Y. (2014). Nutritional intervention for a patient with diabetic nephropathy. *Clinical Nutrition Research, 3*(1), 64–68.

Kirkman, S., Briscoe, V., Clark, N., Florez, H., Hass, L., Halter, J.,...Swift, C. (2012). Diabetes in older adults. *Diabetes Care, 35*(12), 2650-2664.

Leng, S., Tian, X., Matteini, A., Li, H., Hughes, J., Jain, A.,..Fedarko, N. (2011). IL-6-independent association of elevated serum neopterin levels with prevalent frailty in community-dwelling older adults. *Age Ageing, 40*, 475–481.

Liu, K., Lee, W., Liu, L., Chen, L., Lin, M., Peng, L., & Chen, L. (2013). Age-related skeletal muscle mass loss and physical performance in Taiwan: implications to diagnostic strategy of sarcopenia in Asia. *Geriatr Gerontol Int., 13*, 964–971.

López-Otín, C., Blasco, M., Partridge, L., Serrano, M., & Kroemer, G. (2013). The hallmarks of aging. *Cell, 153*(6), 1194–1217. doi: 10.1016/j.cell.2013.05.039

National Institute of Health (2015). *The biology of ageing*. Retrieved from https://www.nia.nih.gov/health/publication/aging-under-microscope/what-aging

Newgard, C., & Pessin, J. (2014). Recent progress in metabolic signaling pathways regulating aging and life span. *J Gerontol A Biol Sci Med Sci., 69*(1), S21–S27.

Onder, G., Cammen, T., Petrovic, M., Somers, A., & Rajkumar, C. (2013). Strategies to reduce the risk of iatrogenic illness in complex older adults. *Age Ageing, 42*(3), 284-291. doi: 10.1093/ageing/aft038

Permpongkosol, S. (2011). Iatrogenic disease in the elderly: risk factors, consequences, and prevention. *Clin Interv Aging, 6*, 77–82. doi: 10.2147/CIA.S10252

Punthakee, Z., Miller, M., Launer, L., ACCORD Group of Investigators, ACCORD-MIND Investigators (2012). Poor cognitive function and risk of severe hypoglycemia in type 2 diabetes: post hoc epidemiologic analysis of the ACCORD trial. *Diabetes Care, 35*, 787–793.

Ramarathan, R., Kohli, A., Ingaramo, M., Jain, A., Leng, S., Punjabi, N.,… Fedarko, N. (2013). Serum chitotriosidase, a putative marker of chronically activated macrophages, increases with normal aging. *J Gerontol A Biol Sci Med Sci., 68*, 1303–1309.

Shang, L., Chen, S., Du, F., Li, S., Zhao, L., & Wang, X. (2011). Nutrient starvation elicits an acute autophagic response mediated by Ulk1 dephosphorylation and its subsequent dissociation from AMPK. *Proc Natl Acad Sci USA, 108*(12), 4788–4793.

YOUR KNOWLEDGE HAS VALUE

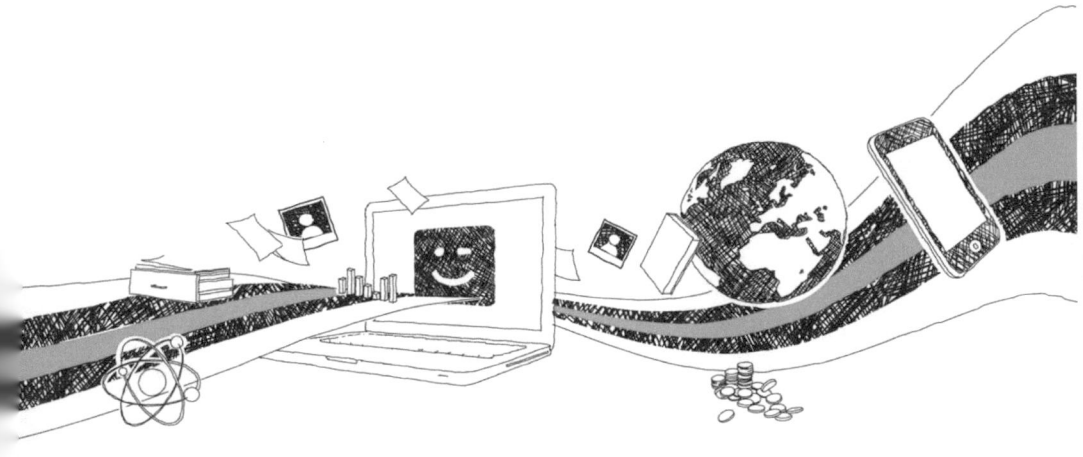

- We will publish your bachelor's and master's thesis, essays and papers

- Your own eBook and book - sold worldwide in all relevant shops

- Earn money with each sale

Upload your text at www.GRIN.com
and publish for free

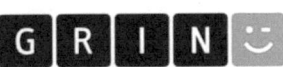